Also by Dr. Stenbeck

Available from the usual on-line source

Books
Healing Yourself -- The Holistic Approach
  [An introduction to Holistic Self-healing.]

Heal Yourself Right Now!
  [The Seven Priority Organ Levels for
  effective Nutritional/Holistic Treatment of
  all organs.]

The 22 Unique Body Types
  (for Health and Weight Loss)
Q & A to Identify Your Body Type (Booklet)
  [Individual Type booklets are also available

Booklets
(Step-by-step instructions on healing yourself)

  #1 Start Healing with Positive Thinking
  #2 Mastering Positive Feelings for Health!
  #3 Spiritual Balance and Your Healing

———

The Nitropheric Body Type

The Ben Affleck, Kate Winslet Celebrity Body Type

For Kaye,
there at the beginning with Doc Severn,
and for Liberty,
continuing the holistic healing journey...

Disclaimer

The information in this book is for educational purposes only and is not a substitute for medication, diets, or other medical care. The diets do not treat diseases or medical conditions, and are an adjunct to your orthodox health care.

The author and publisher accept no responsibility for any misuse of the information within. If you have any physical problem, food allergy, emotional disorder, or disease, common sense dictates that you consult with a physician before changing your diet, taking nutritional supplements, or following the advice given here.

About the Author

Educated in New Zealand and in the U.S.A., Dr. Stenbeck attained B.Sc. (NZ), M.S., and D.C. degrees. His holistic healing methods have been profiled in magazines (Esquire, McLean's, Playgirl, the Atlanta Constitution), and on TV in the USA and in Canada. He was the main contributor to the Warner Book, _The Eye/Body Connection_ by Jessica Maxwell that focused on the holistic healing relationships between the iris structure and organ genetics.

In the 1970-80's he was elected Fellow, Royal Society of Health, London; Fellow, American Association of Chemists; Member, American Association of Clinical Chemists; and Affiliate, Royal Society of Medicine, London. He studied naturopathy and Body Types with Dr. Bernard Jensen and Dr. Clifford Severn, and has practiced in medical partnerships where patients received the joint benefits of medical and holistic healing.

He is a member of Self-Realization Fellowship. To receive advice on any health issue from a holistic viewpoint, or to receive help with your body type, see his web site: *DrStenbeck.net*

———

Contents

* * *

The 22 Types with Celebrity Examples   x
A Succinct Quote from Victor Rocine   xiii
Prologue   xiv

The Nitropheric Body Type (and Food Guide)

   1

Appendix

A. Types / Minerals   58
6. Researchers   61
C. Genetics, Types, and Diet   63
D. Help identifying your body type,
   with Dr. Stenbeck   70
E. On-line Health Consultation
   with Dr. Stenbeck   69
F. Notes   70

* * *

The 22 Body Types:
Celebrity Examples

This Booklet contains the **Nitropheric** *type.
See* <u>*The 22 Unique Body Types*</u> *for all type
descriptions.]*

Thin Types

Atrophic	*Woody Allen / Audrey Hepburn* *Stan Laurel / Calista Flockheart*
Exesthesic	*Cher / Sarah Jessica Parker* *(Female type only)*
Marasmic	*President Obama / Princess Diana* *James Stewart / Kate Blanchard*
Neurogenic	*J.K. Simmons / Joan Rivers* *Jon Cryer / Marin Hinle*
Pathoferic	*(No celebrity males)* *Blythe Danner / Gwyneth Paltrow*
Sillevitic	*David Bowie / Shirley MacLaine* *Rod Stewart / Carol Channing*

Muscle Types

Calciferic	*Michael Jordan / Angelica Huston* *Abrahma Lincoln / Grace Jones*
Carbogenic	*George Clooney / Lady Gaga* *Pres. G. Bush, Jr., Meg Ryan*
Desmogenic	*Marlon Brando / Loni Anderson* *Daniel Craig / Tina Turner*
Eldic	*Ross Perot / Hillary Clinton* *Peter Falk / Sigourney Weaver*
Myogenic	*Pres. Bill Clinton / Sharon Stone* *Pres. John Kennedy / Julia Roberts*
Medeic	*David Caruso / Madonna* *Gary Oldman / Marlene Dietrich*
Nervimotive	*Frank Sinatra / Elizabeth Taylor* *Mark Wahlberg / Natalie Wood*
Nitropheric	*Ben Affleck / Ava Gardner* *Kirk Douglas / Kate Winslet*
Pallinomic	*Pres. Donald Trump /* *Attorney General Janet Reno* *Bill O'Reilly (Fox) / Jane Russell*

Fat Types

Barotic	*Robin Williams / "Mrs. Doubtfire"* *Elton John / William Conrad*
Carboferic	*Bill Murray / Roseanne* *Billy Gardell / Melissa McCarthy*
Hydripheric	*John Goodman / Shelly Winters* *Wayne Knight / Jennifer Holliday*
Isogenic	*Einstein / Oprah Winfrey* *Phillip S. Hoffman / Queen Victoria*
Lipopheric	*Rush Limbaugh / Rosie O'Donnell* *Chris Christie / Camryn Manheim*
Oxypheric	*Winston Churchill / Orsen Welles* *Ella Fitzgerald / Gerry Spence*
Pargenic	*Burt Reynolds / Katey Segal* *Ron Perlman / Kirstey Alley*

Succinct Quote on Human Types

From Victor Rocine, who first described discrete body types around 1900.

"A type is an order of people that differentiates and distinguishes itself by a general and similar form, brain-formation, chemistry, structure, build, immunity, tendencies, predisposition, resemblance, skin-pigment, and type characteristics based on observation and analogy.

"Or, in other words, people of a given type are similar physically and like-minded as if they were brothers and sisters—that is what type means.

"Everything in nature is made according to plan. Man only discovers that plan and gives it a name. The zoologist has not made the animals—he has only described the plan adopted by the wonderful Creator, and named the classes, sub-classes, etc.

"How important type research will be to humanity, time alone will make known."

———

Prologue

The esteemed scientist J. J. Berzelius, discoverer of several chemical elements, inspired Victor Rocine to research body types and to investigate the correlation between types and their diseases. Around 1890-1910, Rocine privately published his original findings on the mineral basis of different body types, and this present book exists because of his brilliant insights.

For many years, I studied with Dr. Clifford Severn who had been a personal student of Victor Rocine on body types, naturopathy, herbology, iris analysis, diet, and nutritional healing methods. He had a successful career as a lecturer and healer, and was one of those rare athletes with complete muscle control over his body. I saw him under a spotlight at 85 years of age, contracting and rippling every individual muscle in his perfectly developed body. Field-Marshal Jan Smuts, the WWII South African Prime Minister, devoted a full chapter of his autobiography to how Severn's healing methods had saved his life. In the 1950's, *Life* magazine did a four-page spread on Severn and his family. Fame he had.

Another Rocine student I studied with, Dr. Bernard Jensen wrote of Rocine's body type research and nutritional methods in his privately published book *The Chemistry of Man*.

This book is deeply rooted in Rocine's original work, and with that of Herbert Shelton, M.D., Ph.D. (at Harvard University in the 1930's). I integrated their research with newer dietary and nervous system data along with celebrity examples of each type, hopefully, making this material easier to digest and more entertaining for the reader.

Gayelord Hauser, another Rocine student I knew, was a celebrated health book author. He wrote a popular book on Rocine's types in the 1940's *Types and Temperaments;* reputedly, he also introduced yogurt to the western world.

This book exists because of Rocine's creative brilliance and original discoveries.

▶ *Rocine: "The soul creates the body type."*

Rocine taught that the soul chooses a body type and brain to live in, thus presenting different experiences and life lessons to master. Why were *you* born the way you are?

That is something to think about, especially if it is true! What would your soul purpose be to live in a particular body type. I provide some thoughts on this issue in each type description and try to assess from my experience with your type the particular lessons of life presented therein.

Rocine was as brilliant in his way as an Abraham Lincoln, Michael Jordan, Michael Phelps, Tony Robbins, or a Daniel Day Lewis—all *calciferics*—rare, leaders, innovative, brilliant, and highly intelligent in their different fields of endeavor.

Celebrity examples exist for most types, not a duplicate of you, but someone who has your essence in their body-mind individuality. Knowing your type allows you to become a better you!

The celebrity examples provide further help in identifying your body type.

▶ *Rocine's classic findings are the backbone of this book. Integrated with Sheldon's research and with other dietary and food issues including mental, emotional, and spiritual attributes,*

Many people take nutritional supplements and try different diets without a doctor's advice. If this is your choice, use common sense, listen to body responses, and discontinue any allergic reactions to foods or nutritional substances.

———

The Nitropheric Body Type

Representing one of the 22 Body Types first described by Victor Rocine around 1900

* * *

"You may also have a physical or psychological feature not representaiive of your type such as height, weight, appearance, talent, weakness, strength, etc., due to biochemical errors, environmental influences, racial or cultural differences, and congenital or genetic issues. Nevertheless, the type identification in the average person is usually clear."

— *Victor Rocine*

Nitropheric Type Celebrity Examples

If you think this is your type, be sure to look at **on-line photographs** *of these examples. Look for general similarities to yourself. Note that subtypes cause the differences in appearance between members of the same type.*

ROYALTY

Duke of Edinburgh
Charles, Prince of Wales
Duke of Windsor (King Edward VII)

POLITICS [Many politicians]

President Franklin Roosevelt
President Ronald Reagan
President Gerald Ford
Dick Chenney   Donald Rumsfeld
Nelson Mandela   Anwar Sadat
Dan Quayle   Mitt Romney

MILITARY

General Omar Bradley (WWII)

ACTORS

Ben Affleck

Christopher Plummer

Ralph Fiennes

Joseph Fiennes

Harrison Ford

Denzel Washington

Leonardo di Caprio

Jeff Bridges

William Holden

Robert Vaughn

Treat Williams

John Gavin

Keifer Sutherland

Hal Holbrook

Larry Hagman

Lee Majors

William Hurt

John Forsythe

Jack Hawkins

Walter Pidgeon

Randolph Scott

Treat Williams

John Houseman

Beau Bridges

Alan Bates

John Thaw

River Phoenix

Tom Tryon

Kevin Costner

Anthony Hopkins

George Peppard

William Shatner

James Garner

Brad Pitt

Lloyd Bridges

Leslie Nielsen

Kenneth Branagh

Martin Sheen

Robert Loggia

James Franciscus

John Clease

Danny Glover

Stewart Granger

Spencer Tracy

Arthur Hill

Tyrone Power

Eddie Albert

Nelson Eddy

Jeff Daniels

Sam Neil

Ed Asner

Glen Ford

Terence Stamp

Kenneth More

Chevy Chase

Martin Milner

Patrick McGoohan (BBC: "The Prisoner")

And the beautiful women...

Kate Winslet	Renee Zellweger
Liv Ullmann	Ingrid Bergman
Lana Turner	Jessica Lange
Greer Garson	Kim Novak
Kate Nelligan	Ursula Andress
Marilyn Monroe	Ava Gardner
Deborah Kerr	Veronica Lake
Ginger Rogers	Sophia Loren
Catherine Zeta-Jones	Barbara Eden
And many more!	

(There are examples galore of excellent believable actors with many academy awards. Mostly are of medium-height, a few tall examples.)

MUSIC

Andrea Bocelli	Julio Iglessias
Benny Goodman	Bill Evans (piano)
Nat King Cole	Glen Miller
Benny Goodman	Natalie Cole
Vanilla Ice	

(and many musicians and big band leaders)

TV/ PERSONALITIES

Peter Graves	Walter Cronkite
Peter Jennings	Jim Lampley
Brian Williams	Charles Gibson
Walt Disney	Mike Farrell

Diane Sawyer   Barbara Walters
Jane Pauley   Rick Steves (Travel)
David Brinkley

SPORT

Dan Marino   Mark Langston
Anna Kournikova (tennis)

Many professional and world-class athletes, Olympic tennis and soccer players, are this type: intelligent, high muscle coordination, delicate movements, speed, etc.

OTHE

Charles Lindberg
Dr. Scott-Peck (psychologist)

[Note: I personally knew two of the above celebrities, and many other examples in everyday life and in my family, which contributed to my understanding of the type.

You already know something about this type from their public persona and appearance, whether from seeing them yourself or from the celebrity examples. Blend such insights with the type descriptions and the types of your family and friends to discern their presence in your midst!

Read the types, and if still confused you may choose to use the personal request for type identification from my web site: *DrStenbeck.net*

———

Nitropheric Type Questionnaire

Other than for the physical descriptions, these questions describe the generic type, and not specifically you! If any question ever applied to you, then choose he True answer!

For Question 1 only:

    A = True   *B = Maybe*   *C = Untrue*

    15 points   7 points   1 point

1. Physically identify with celebrity example____

Then…

    A = True   *B = Maybe*   *C = Untrue*

    5 points   3 points   1 point

---

2. Height is close to:
   Males: 5'8-6'5   Females: 5'5-5'10   ____
3. Usual weight is close to:
   Males: 150-230+ Females: 130-175+   ____
4. Body medium-sized, hold fat with age   ____
5. Muscles medium or larger-sized, and moderate strength   ____
6. Luxuriant, soft, wavy, attractive, brown hair (some black); hair thins after age 40 in many males   ____
7. Have a reclusive and refined nature   ____
8. Prominent attractive cheeks; relatively wide cheek bones (not sunken)   ____

9. A fat padding appears under the chin   _____
10. Males handsome; females pretty, lovely, or beautiful, depending upon sub-type   _____
11. Aristocratic and exclusive tastes   _____
12. Teeth white, medium-strength, shapely   _____
13. Tranquil, placid unless provoked   _____
14. Once provoked, decisions based on deep feelings   _____
15. Sensitive to injustice, false accusation   _____
16. Most male sparse, slight chest hair); females medium to large bust   _____
17. Conservative and poised   _____
18. Mentally strong, intellectual potential   _____
19. Regal, noble bearing (know are different to others)   _____
20. Head and face handsome, attractive   _____
21. Forehead square or rectangular shape   _____
22. Attractive eyes, mostly brown (some blue); eyebrows invariably black   _____
23. Males: "humanitarian" forehead lines; females show fine facial lines   _____
24. Mouth and lips lovely   _____
25. Excellent ability to influence others   _____
26. Usually have high intelligence   _____
27. Decisions based on deep feelings not on rational thinking (particularly females)   _____
28. Hips, thighs, abdomen often hold fat   _____
29. Gesture little when speaking   _____
30. Joints, ligaments, tendons weak, easily damaged through athletic injuries   _____

31. Upper arms larger, tapering towards delicate wrists, narrow hands; thighs thicker, narrower lower legs _____
32. Intelligent with executive, leadership, military, and teaching abilities _____
33. Deepest loving feelings are hidden, and voiced with difficulty _____
34. Appear serene, poised, relaxed (even if are not) _____
35. Like to be in-command and in-control _____
36. Physically and emotionally sensitive _____
37. Crave a life of peace, quiet, happiness, and wisdom _____
38. Live truth, allow no compromise to ethics, moral compass and spirituality _____
39. Vulnerable to health problems from chemical, metal toxins (especially females) _____
40. Highly romantic, sentimental; the ladies crave these values in mates _____
41. Feel intensely (anger, love, hate, etc.) _____
42. Desire honesty, justice, honor _____
43. Voice pleasant, impressive, low-toned _____
44. Diplomatic unless irritated; able to reject opponent's viewpoint outright (yet retain their friendship) _____
45. Very loving; need an understanding mate _____
46. Forceful in disciplining children _____
47. Cannot tolerate uninvited familiarity _____
48. Assertive or aggressive _____

49. Dislike physical labor or jobs needing strength, danger, risk, dirt, or heat _____
50. Dislike living alone _____
51. Some females are aloof to other women; males are charming, but some are chauvinistic or macho _____
52. Females: other women competitive and jealous of you; males: other types are competitive of your "all American" appearance _____
53. Excellent memory for sentiments (tend to live in the past) _____
54. Thoughtful and deliberate courage _____
55. Crave independence; females may depend on others _____
56. Tend to grant favors and permission beyond what is appropriate (good will may be taken advantage of) _____
57. Have self-composure and self-control _____
58. Believe in discipline, law, order, truth _____
59. Appreciate antiquity and history _____
60. Often are controlling in relationships _____
61. May be sarcastic if provoked _____
62. Easily forgive and excuse own negative behaviors _____
63. Strong rivalry and jealousy sense _____
64. Is unrewarding to argue with you (the mind is ruled by sentiments, not by rational thoughts; mostly females) _____
65. May be excessively outspoken _____
66. If insulted, show calm, but the offender may pay _____

67. Dislike being rushed: follow your own schedule _____

68. Tardy tendency, may be late for appointments and keep others waiting _____

69. May be attracted to metaphysics, conspiracy, psychics, etc. _____

Scoring

For Question #1:
A response: give 15 points = _____
B response: give 7 points = _____
C response: give 1 points = _____

For Questions #2—69:
A response: give 5 points = _____
B response: give 3 points = _____
C response: give 1 point = _____

Total of the above points = _____

Interpretation
187—325 PROBABLY Nitropheric type
95—186: POSSIBLY Nitropheric type
<95: NOT Nitropheric type

The Nitropheric Type

Rocine: "Nitropheric means 'nitrogen carrying'.
Nitrogen in nature is inert, and likewise, it
parallels inertness and exclusivity as key
aspectsof your personality. You utilize more food
nitrogen than other types." You are poised,
refined, aristocratic, and highly emotionally
sensitive.

———

E motionally hidden, exclusive, serene, and noble in bearing are qualities that characterize your type. You are medium-sized, with some tending to become heavier with age (due to a fat sub-type, often *carboferic*). Careful dieting and exercising maintains your health and weight control. One variety of your type, for example, is invariably heavier from mid-teens onwards, as in the Bridges acting family: father Lloyd is medium-sized, Jeff is tall and medium-sized, and Beau fights the fat (invariably due to a fat sub-type).

► *Rocine: "You are largely unknowable, your*
emotions being deep and secret. Others may see
you as cold and distant, but in fact, you are
highly emotionally sensitive. You have difficulty
expressing this sensitivity."

These characteristics make you emotion-laden Oscar worthy actors like Anthony Hopkins, Ben Affleck, Ralph Fiennes, Gregory Peck, Jessica Lange, Kim Novak, and Greer Garson.

Genetically, you are born to be a partial vegetarian, highlighting your greatest health problem: excessive flesh eating. For health, you need more vegetable proteins and alkaline-ash foods (fruits, salads, and vegetables) with less acid-ash foods (flesh and carbohydrates, especially beef). (A carnivorous sub-type modifies this recommendation allowing more flesh).

———

Physical Similarity to Other Types

The medium-sized *carbogenic* type (Sally Field, Alec Baldwin) is handsome or attractive, and medium-sized when younger.

The male *myogenic* type (President Clinton, Julia Roberts) is attractive, lean or medium-sized.

The *desmogenic* type (Marlon Brando, Loni Anderson) is medium-sized when young, although often larger with age.

The *pallinomic* type (John Wayne, Esther Williams) is muscular and medium when young, but carries much solid fat with aging.

———

Average Height and Weight

Males:	5'8-6'5	150-230+ pounds
Females:	5'5-5'10	130-175+ pounds

———

Nitropheric Type Description

The type description represents how you appear in everyday society. You may have a sub-type that alters parts of this description.

Think of the celebrity examples as you read the descriptions. You are an attractive muscular type, of medium-height with some taller males, while the females, particularly, have a fat-making tendency. Your proportional body may become heavier with age (from a fat sub-type).

You are shapely and lovely women, some-what fatty over the hips and pelvis, upper arms and thighs. Marilyn Monroe exemplifies the sensual, medium-sized woman of your type, such women often being beautiful (Sophia Loren, Greer Garson, Jessica Lange, Kim Novak). The men are often handsome as in Harrison Ford,

Gregory Peck, Brad Pitt, Ben Affleck, William Holden.

Head —Your head and face are balanced and pleasing in appearance. The forehead is high, square, or rectangular-shaped. Your face is full, attractive, handsome, or beautiful with medium-sized cheekbones.

▶ *Rocine: "If female, you are the most highly sentimental type. It is useless to argue with you, as one can never argue with a sentiment nor reason with a feeling—you feel your truth and that is that! One can reason with the mind of most types, but not with your feelings!"*

[If spiritually evolved you may sometimes change your mind; the males have a rational mind to neutralize this emotional issue.]

Hair — You have lovely, wavy, soft, glossy, luxuriant, attractive, and brown hair (some black); with aging the males show a slight or moderate hair loss tendency (from the temples backwards).

Eyes — Your eyes are usually brown or blue; the eyebrows often black.

Ears — Your ears tend to be normal and shapely, some smaller than average, or larger due to an *eldic* sub-type.

Nose — A normal or smaller-sized nose is usual, some are thin and longer.

Face —Typically, you have a shapely face with gently curving and wide facial bones. You seldom show facial wrinkles, but have "humanitarian" lines across the forehead (males usually). A fatty padding may arise under your chin with aging. Your facial expression and feelings are hidden until you express them explosively—then everyone look out (especially if you have a *desmogenic* sub-type, which is quite common)!

► *If male, you are invariably attractive or handsome. You often work-out and are muscular and strong; your muscles and joints are of average strength (but with a desmogenic or carbogenic sub--type you may be very strong).*

Mouth and Lips —Your mouth and lips are normal-sized, shapely, lovely, inviting, with the upper lip often larger in the center. Your lips may be beautiful and inviting, the lower lip full and shapely. The voice is sweet and charming, but if upset you may be caustic and demanding without realizing or caring that your tone of voice is hurting the feelings of others. As actors, you have impressive speaking voices.

Teeth — Your teeth and calcium metabolism are strong and attractive.

Skin — You may have a somewhat olive-complexion; the hair and eyes are usually darker.

Neck — The neck is medium-sized, or may be shorter, muscular, and thicker if overweight.

Muscles — You fill the health clubs, working out and looking good, but are not usually found in endurance sports or work requiring great strength. You are a mental person of average strength with excellent brain and limb coordination that allows excellence in sports like tennis, soccer, polo, baseball, and dancing, but never boxing. A muscular sub-type allows greater strength.

Chest — Your chest is large and deep. The men typically have a light chest hair growth, but exceptions do occur (with a *carbogenic, nervimotive, or pargenic* sub-type).

▶ *The bust is medium to large with some beautiful Playboy centerfolds being of your type. (Note that most centerfolds and fashion models are myogenics with breast augmentation.)*

Back and Shoulders —The back and shoulders are markedly muscular; the females have a graceful and elegant back.

Hips and Abdomen —The hips and abdomen are vulnerable to holding excessive fat; if male you may show a pot belly by age 40-45. Exercise and diet are essential for keeping your figure (daily walking is the best exercise for females).

Arms and Legs —Your upper arms are larger, tapering towards delicate wrists and hands; you have thick thighs with narrower lower legs.

▶ *You gesture little when speaking impulsively, and are uncomfortable moving your arms and hands—you make natural actors: you appear to have superb self-control under stress. Actually, you are as nervous as anyone else!*

Joints —Weak and vulnerable joints, ligaments and tendons are easily hurt through athletic injuries.

———

Nitropheric Personality Traits

If you are this Muscle type many, but not all, of the following characteristics are present (you may have overcome or moderated the negatives, but should recognize that you once had several of them.

You may have any of the following traits:

- Romantic and sentimental
- Excellent networking ability
- Don't confide easily in strangers
- Are loyal and hospitable to friends
- May possess a wry sense of humor
- May be expert in art, antiques, history
- Are physically and emotionally sensitive
- Others are magnetically attracted to you
- Have high self-confidence and self-image
- Crave peace and quiet, happiness, wisdom
- Assertive and aggressive; low raw courage
- Exclusive, intelligent, poised, and refined
- Vulnerable to low self: esteem, self-love
- Live your truth, right or wrong (no compromise)
- Feelings and sentiments are deeply hidden
- Have qualities of high self-composure and self-control

- Great judges of dress, deportment, fashion, elegance
- Have strong sense of reverence, honor, modesty, trust
- Excellent memory for past sentiments, and hurts by others
- Have hidden innermost feelings (except for closest friends)
- Feel very deeply and intensely: whether love or hate; disciplinarian
- Like to influence others; high belief in law, order, discipline, truth
- Are able to reject outright an opponents viewpoint yet retain their friendship
- Will not respond to the expectations of others: follow the beat of your own drummer
- Intense dislikes for: living alone, selfish people, being rushed, and being misunderstood
- Like to be in command; have high leadership skills; are born leaders (and strategic generals)
- Strong in honesty, justice, honor, principle: will quit a highly paid job if principle demands it
- Always look calm, in control, serene, unruffled, poised, relaxed, even if not (until intense stress causes you to lose it)

▶ *Rocine:* *"You appear to others as being lordly and perfect in your own eyes, but nevertheless you discredit yourself and may feel no self-confidence. Others don't know this, but you do!"*

Potential Challenges

You may have evolved from or not experienced these faults so do not dwell on them:

- Cannot tolerate familiarity
- May be very sarcastic if irritated
- Difficulty in expressing deep love
- Tend to crave money and affluence
- High sense of litigation when wronged
- Have fears of the future, disease, poverty
- Dislike and do not manage change well
- Some have self: sabotage, destruction
- If female, other female types are jealous of you
- Easily feel misunderstood by loved ones or spouses
- Like to stay up late, and to sleep late in the morning
- May have negative habit patterns that are hard to break

- Have an intense, strong, negative, and fearful imagination
- May be late for appointments, and keep others waiting (especially females)
- Strongly developed in rivalry, jealousy, criticism, competitiveness, and in needing to control others
- Forgive and excuse own negative behaviors too easily (and rarely say, or mean, "I'm sorry")
- High opinion of self, sometimes excessively so; tendency to be aloof, distant and detached
- Females may be dependent on others: this is a type challenge to become independent and autonomous
- Tendency to allow, forgive, permit, agree, be naïve, and grant favors and permission too easily (for which you may be easily hurt)

▶ *If you relate to any of these challenges, doing something to overcome them serves your evolution.*

———

Nitropheric Stress Management

You have strong mental stress prevention giving you a good ability not to internalize this stress into your stomach, adrenals, and immune system. When highly stressed you need affirmations and nerve nutrition. Emotional stress prevention is not strong, and the above challenges may need repro-gramming. (You benefit by following the advice in Booklets #1 and 2.).

————

Love

You ache for a loving relationship, but rarely trust a loved one enough to feel safe communicating deep loving feelings. The males have difficulty expressing love unless blessed with a sensitive nature (or sub-type); they are charming, but some may become chauvinistic. You are often attracted to the *carbogenic, carboferic, desmogenic, myogenic, nervimotive, and pathoferic* types. Your sexual drive is medium to strong, and under the right circumstances, you may be intensely aroused.

▶ *Rocine: "At the end of his life, a man married to a nitropheric lady still does not know if she really loved him." (Likewise, for a woman married to a nitropheric man. Of course, an evolved nitropheric moderates their judgmental nature, and learns to expresses their deep loving feelings.)*

————

Talents and Vocations

Abilities - *Executive, leadership, military, politics, teaching*

When others put your talents to work in the right business, you come into your own and accomplish your goals.

You are intelligent and highly talented with strong and often unrealized ambitions. You dream about doing great things, but may be unmotivated. Many of you work in medicine, science, engineering, and teaching.

You should work where your honesty and trustworthiness is appreciated. An example is America's most trusted broadcaster of the past, Walter Cronkite, who was noble, honest, ethical, trustworthy, reserved, intelligent, and talented. Other *nitropheric* examples are Peter Jennings and Barbara Walters (and most successful TV anchors). The males, particularly, are born to leadership: General Omar Bradley, an excellent example, who brought great leadership and intelligence to helping win World War II. Bradley, supervised by General Dwight Eisenhower *(neurogenic)* worked under General Marshall *(nitropheric);* who worked for President Roosevelt *(myogenic)*, who ran the war with Winston Churchill *(oxypheric)* and Joseph Stalin *(desmogenic)*. President Truman *(eldic)* ordered the dropping of the Atomic Bomb on Japan in 1945.

▶ *I have seen you successful in: teaching, holistic healing, the stock market, in academics (sciences, engineering), and particularly in medicine.*

Generally, you have a good sporting ability, with stars in baseball, tennis, and soccer. The type information cannot predict what or who you will become, but you are capable of bringing a creative excellence or brilliance to your life.

Inabilities - *Physical labor*
You dislike work in dirty surroundings or any position requiring risk, danger, physical strength, or temperature extremes.

———

Nitropheric Health Problems

Your type has low vitality and constitutional strength. Generally, your organs and tissues are sensitive and vulnerable to becoming unhealthy, unless you take preventive action to heal yourself. You commonly experience problems in any of the following systems:

Heart — The heart and vascular system is weak (and made worse by eating beef).

Toxicity — Your organs readily retain environmental toxic metals, chemicals, and free radicals, for which nutrition is needed.

Intestines — Your intestines are genetically weak and liable to constipation; having enemas and colonic irrigation helps.

▶ *The females are unusually vulnerable to health problems from chemical, metal, and toxic substances in foods and the environment: holistic healing is essential for you. I have had female patients of this type (and the atrophic type) who could not live in modern homes because of their sensitivity to electromagnetic fields, chemicals in carpeting and upholstery, etc.*

Mind — Excess nitrogen in your diet makes you more secretive, inhibited, dreamy, and passive.

———

Acid/Alkaline Factor

[See the Appendix for details on this subject, along with the common symptoms found with people of different nervous system dominance.]

For your health and healing, the genetics of your autonomic nervous system predispose you to needing a specific ratio of food acidity to alkalinity. Your acid constitution requires a mostly **alkaline-ash** diet for acid/alkaline balance. (Ash refers to minerals left in your body after metabolizing foods.) Your nervous system genetics are *sympathetic* dominant.

Construct this approximate ratio of daily food selections:

> *70% Fruits, salads, vegetables*
> *30% Proteins, carbohydrates*

▶ *Approximate your food ratios. On any particular day, it does not matter if one meal is mostly alkaline and another mostly acid—just try to balance it out for the day! If you make a mistake, try again tomorrow. It is a subjective call that you make, and what is done over time that makes the difference to your health.*

————

The Nitropheric Spiritual Factor

Skip this paragraph if uninterested in a philosophical perspective on your type!

▶ *Rocine: "The soul chooses the body type."*

If as souls, we choose the brain and body type to spend a lifetime in, it could be to learn certain spiritual lessons related to perfecting ourselves, and our humanity, in God's eyes. What lessons does the type bring you? Only you can really decide what those lessons are. You know your weaknesses, faults, and behaviors towards others. You know things about yourself that Victor Rocine could never get from his research subjects when he first wrote about types. So search your mind for the answers.

Each discrete type has challenges of life lessons, spiritual goals, etc., and some of yours may be:

God Relationship — The males, particularly, may feel separated from God: read spiritual books, go to church, find your faith, and you will become more loving and friendly.

Co-dependency — Becoming independent and autonomous is a challenge for the females.

Controlling — You tend to be controlling in relationships (although you may deny it); the males may be "macho", for which counseling is helpful (particularly in a marriage).

Deep Fears — You have many fears; counseling and spirituality are helpful.

Excessive Self-forgiveness — You forgive and excuse your own negative behaviors too easily: ease up and be more humble!

Difficulty Expressing Love — Your loved ones may never know whether they are really loved:

allow yourself to hug, be affectionate, and express love at every opportunity! It is too easy for you to sit on your laurels and assume you are doing enough in relationships.

Attractiveness — Your soul chose to live in a shapely feminine or handsome body. How has that served your growth and evolution?

———

A Nitropheric Story...

Veronica, age 34, a lovely woman with a radiant personality complained of a steadily increasing weight problem. Examination showed her to be healthy except for a sub-clinical toxic liver problem that required herbal detoxifying. She had no medical problems.

She had liver-kidney inefficiency and water-weight due to excessive intake of flesh foods: meats, poultry, fish, and eggs. (Instead, she needed more legumes, peas, beans, black-eyed peas, seeds, nuts, and pasta.) In addition, there was a tissue acidity problem from excessive eating of <u>cooked</u> sulfur foods: cabbage, onions, cauliflower, garlic, Brussels sprouts, broccoli, and mustard greens. There was also a key deficit in calcium, an important mineral for her type, and she needed two daily servings of foods, like kelp, Swiss and cheddar cheese, turnip greens, almonds, and parsley.

Veronica made the needed dietary changes, took supplemental calcium, and her weight steadily decreased as she returned to and maintained her optimum weight.

———

Nitropheric Type Mineral Foods

Apply this mineral data to the diet following these Muscle type descriptions.

Excessive Foods:

- *Nitrogen (beef)*
- *Carbon (simple carbohydrates)*
- *Sulfur (cooked)*
- *Sodium (salted, junk)*

Deficient Foods:

- *Calcium (very important)*
- *Nitrogen (non-beef, vegetable)*
- *Sodium (unsalted, non-junk))*
- *Sulfur (raw)*
- *Magnesium*
- *Trace Minerals*

These deficient nutrients are common deficiencies in your type and predispose you to ill-health. If ill, be sure to use these lists with your <u>daily</u> food intake. If not ill, eat from the foods lists 3-4 times <u>weekly</u>. All food lists are in descending order of concentration and value to you; choose servings of foods in the upper half of each list first! One serving is ½ cup.

Nitropheric Excessive Foods -

Nitrogen from red meat is excessive in your diet (if eaten more than once monthly) and is a major cause of your acidity and illnesses; poultry, fish, and eggs should be limited to three days weekly with vegetarian proteins like legumes (peas, beans), seeds, nuts and pasta on the other days. Your genetics require a vegetarian, semi-vegetarian (or vegan) diet.

Carbon is excessive in your type. It is excessive in all people who become fat or obese, and is found in every cell of the body as the basis of life. You need to avoid white sugar foods, simple carbohydrates, corn syrups (or fat will accumulate).

Sulfur in <u>cooked</u> form is excessive in your tissues bringing excess sulfur acids into your tissues with toxicity and emotional instability.

Sodium from salted junk foods is excessive in your tissues. To preserve your health and weight control avoid junk foods, and fulfill your sodium needs from the food list (without using the salt- shaker).

———

Deficient Foods –

In illness or disease, it is important to correct these mineral deficiencies.

Calcium is often deficient in your type, and you thrive on dairy foods. It is highly concentrated in bones, joints, muscles, nerves, heart, teeth, and gums; if you have an illness or disease in any of these tissues, calcium foods and supplements are often a significant healing factor.

Nitrogen from vegetable sources is deficient (see above notes).

Sodium from unsalted foods is deficient (see above note).

Sulfur from raw food sources is deficient.

Magnesium may be deficient; it is important for heart, digestive function.

Trace minerals easily become deficient due to emotional stress or poor digestion and absorption. *[See the Appendix for descriptive notes on minerals.]*

Minimize
Excessive Mineral Foods

Nitrogen (beef): *0-1 servings/<u>month</u>*
Beef, red meats

Carbon, Sodium (salted, junk):
0-1 servings/<u>week</u>

Grains, breads, sweet fruits, white sugar foods, sugars, fats, salt, all fast foods, packaged foods, canned and frozen foods, soy sauce, all preserved meats (cured, smoked, canned and luncheon meats), sauces (barbecue, catsup, etc.), dill pickles, sauerkraut, bouillon cubes, peanut butter, potato chips, etc., salted nuts, crackers, canned or packaged soups, processed cheeses, commercial salad dressings.

Sulfur (cooked): *0-1 servings/week*

Cabbage, onions, cauliflower, Brussels sprouts, garlic, broccoli, turnips, mustard greens, rutabagas, and spinach.

Note: If you must eat anything on the above lists, keep it down to ½ cup, weekly!

<u>Eat</u>

Deficient Mineral Foods

Nitrogen (vegetable):

Legumes, peas, beans, black-eyed peas, seeds, nuts, pasta, spirulina, and tofu
    1-2 servings/day
Poultry, fish, eggs ——0-3 times/week

Sodium (unsalted, non-junk):
    1-2 servings/day

Kelp, scallops, blue and goat's cheese, goat's milk, strawberries, Swiss chard, coconut, beets and greens, lentils, nuts, oats, okra, poultry and gizzards, celery, salt water fish, sesame seeds.

Sulfur (raw):
    1-2 servings/day

Cauliflower, cabbage, onions, garlic, spinach, figs, carrots, hors-radish, radishes, almonds, chestnuts, oranges, shrimp

Eat

Deficient foods...

Calcium, Magnesium:
1-2 servings/day
Kelp, Swiss and cheddar cheese, almonds, cashews, blackstrap molasses, brewer's yeast, buckwheat, parsley, dandelion greens, brazil nuts, watercress, tofu, dulse, filberts, peanuts, millet, pecan.

Trace Minerals : 1-2 servings/day

Kelp, goat's cheese and milk, raw garlic, sprouts, rhubarb, beet greens, peach, alfalfa, ginger, rice, oats, pineapples, dry split peas, blackstrap molasses, seeds, nuts, brown rice, oat straw tea.
Note: Eat any healthy foods you desire, but be sure to include the type foods in your daily choices.

Note -

The recommendations here are for the generic type. Additionally, you may need from a holistic healer or nutritionist something more specific for your individuality.

Nitropheric Nutritional Supplements

- **Multi-Minerals** —*[Take all supplements with food]*
  2 capsules/day

- **Calcium** —*Important!*
  600 mg/twice daily (with betaine hydrochloride)

- **Herbs** —
  Brain detox – Chickweed or Valerian Rt.
  Organ detox – Milk Thistle or Strawberry Leaf
  (Take one capsule, twice daily for one month; then one capsule, three times weekly.)

- **Lecithin** —
  About 1,300 mg/three times weekly

- **Evening Primrose or Flaxseed Oil**
  1 soft-gel/day

- **If Vegetarian** —
  Be sure to take a protein drink daily.

- **Other** — *Take as directed: three times weekly, of chlorella, chlorophyll, blue-green algae, green magma, spirulina, alfalfa.*

Important Nitropheric Health Concerns

Your nervous system genetics require the *Vegetarian (or Semi-vegetarian)* Food Guide for health. Unlike other muscle types, you have weak carnivorous genes. Any vegetarian leanings are healthy for you, and red meats should be restricted to once monthly (which may be difficult for you).

▶ *Rocine: "You become over-acid and sick from excessive intake of animal nitrogen, starches, carbohydrates, and cooked sulfur foods. Dairy and calcium foods (and supplements) are essential for your health and healing."*

Some of you appear to be lactose deficient, requiring that you also take lactase tablets with dairy foods.

You are usually sensitive to chemical preservatives, gluten, white sugar, drugs, caffeine, alcohol, wheat, cocoa, and GMO foods; remove such allergic foods from your diet.

<u>*Nitropheric Food Guide*</u>

Aim for -

70% Fruits, salads, vegetables
30% Proteins, complex carbohydrates
and
70% Raw food diet
30% Cooked foods

Avoid cooked sulfur foods.
Eat calcium and dairy foods.
Note Rocine's comments.
Eat the recommended supplements.

Nitropheric Weight Loss

Around 1900, Rocine wrote that you are a Fat type, but now in modern times I see you mostly as a Muscle type (who can easily gain fat). You gain weight easily, but it is relatively easily lost compared to the classic Fat types who struggle intensely to burn fat. In modern times, mostly, you eat and exercise sensibly, and you look like mesomorphs.

The males seldom have weight problems, easily addressed by reducing calorie intake; for the females, it is more different. Losing weight depends upon you following the type instructions, summarized in this section.

- *Gluten* is often an allergic factor
- *Stop* eating junk carbon and sodium foods
- *Protein* drink daily, have about 25-30 grams
- *Eat* your body type deficient mineral foods daily
- *Gluten:* a common allergy; remove it from your diet
- *Follow* your *Nitropheric Guide (as above)*
- *Exercise:* your body type requires moderate daily exercise (walking or jogging is excellent)
- *Simple sugars:* stop all white table sugar and high-fructose corn syrup and drinks containing these sugars
- *Hypoglycemia:* this hormonal imbalance stops fat loss, and usually initiates more fat production, so it is vital to deal with this problem if it affects you: take *pantothenic acid,* 500 mg/twice daily with food (see my earlier books to resolve this problem)
- *Calories:* As with any dietary approach, calories in, must be *less than* calories out! Most markets sell a calorie booklet; make notes of your daily intake, and in most instances keep it under about 1500 calories/dav

———

Nitropheric Type
General Food Guide

Vegetarian (or Semi-)

Important Note

―――

The Food Guide addresses the <u>Acid-Alkaline</u> aspect of your food intake, along with the <u>Type Mineral</u> factor presented throughout this book. It does <u>not</u> necessarily address calories or other dietary factors that may be pertinent to your personal health needs whether medical or appropriate for some other dietary need. So use your common sense and just include the factors described here with whatever healthy dietary choices you usually make.

For other nutrient information, consult with nutritional books or with holistic nutritional doctors. I particularly recommend the advice of Andrew Weil, M.D.

―――

General Food Guide

This chapter presents a general Food Guide, upon which you superimpose the nutritional information from your type chapter.

Meat/Flesh Intake

Most muscle types should limit red meat to once or less weekly, while eggs, lamb, fish, or poultry are excellent in moderation. If ill or diseased, be sure to eat daily, one or two servings from each *deficient minerals* list. If not ill, eat them at least three times weekly for health maintenance. If this diet is similar to your present diet, but healing is sluggish, then:

- Decrease your carbohydrate and protein intake by about one-third
- Increase your fruit, salad, and vegetable intake by about one-third
- Consult with a holistic doctor, preferably one versed in nutritional and emotional evaluation

---

Over-Acid or Over-Alkaline?

Just as a log of wood burned in your fireplace leaves a mineral-ash, food ash refers to the minerals remaining after metabolizing foods in your tissues:

- Fruits, vegetables **alkalinize** tissues
- Proteins, carbohydrates **acidify** tissues

Usually You Are Over-Acid Due To:

- Excessive intake of dairy foods
- Excessive intake of proteins and carbohydrates
- Deficient intake of fruits, salads and vegetables
- Accumulated metabolic waste-acids (from years of eating excessive acid-ash foods, meats and carbohydrates, and from lack of exercise)
- You need to estimate the ratio of foods eaten. Generally, eat the following *approximate* ratios for your health:

70% <u>Alkaline-ash</u> foods *(fruits, salads, vegetables)*

30% <u>Acid-ash</u> foods *(complex carbo-hydrates like starches, grains, cereals, breads, flour products; and proteins)*

Approximate your food ratios. On any particular day, it does not matter if one meal is mostly alkaline, and another mostly acid—just try to balance it out for the day! If you get it wrong, try again tomorrow. It is a subjective call that you make, and it is what you do over weeks, months, or years that make the difference—not on any one or two days.

———

Important

- Minimize white sugar and alcohol intake.
- If desired, interchange lunches for dinners.
- Never eat foods you are allergic to, no matter what I recommend; if allergic, or suspect a food allergy, eliminate it and substitute from your type mineral lists.
- Eat the right foods 80-90% of the time and the Food Guide will work for you; unlike some types you do not have to live out of a health food store (although such foods are healthier for you).

▶ *Omit eating the excessive minerals in your type chapter, and be sure to eat one or two servings from the deficient list daily.*

Finally, in addition to your body type needs, other holistic healing matters also need your attention. I strongly suggest that you refer to my web site and earlier books for that information: *DrStenbeck.net*

———

On any particular day, it does not matter if one meal is mostly alkaline, and another mostly acid—just try to balance it out for the day! If you make a mistake, try again tomorrow. It is a subjective call that you make, and it is what you do over weeks, months, or years that make the difference—not on any one or two days or weeks.

———

Acid/Alkaline Genetics, Dietary-Ash, and Raw Food Needs

This chart shows the Rocine types, their acid or alkaline food needs, and the percentage of raw foods needed for your health and healing.

- Apply this Chart and Type Minerals to the Food Guide

Type	Acid/Alkaline Genetics	% Food-Ash Needed	% Raw Food Needed
Calciferic	Alkaline	70% acid	30
Carbogenic	Alkaline	50-50	50
Desmogenic	Alkaline	70% acid	50
Eldic	Intermediate	50-50	50
Medeic	Intermediate	50-50	50
Myogenic	Intermediate	50-50	50
Nervimotive	Alkaline	70% acid	50
Nitropheric	Acid	70% _alkaline_	70
Pallinomic	Alkaline	50-50	30

The above percentages vary depending on aging and the health of individual types.

▶ *Observe the excessive minerals in your type chapter, and be sure to eat one or two servings from the deficient list daily (or, several times weekly).*

———

Important

- Minimize white sugar and alcohol intake.

- If desired, interchange lunches for dinners.

- Never eat foods you are allergic to no matter what is recommended; if allergic or suspect a food allergy, eliminate it and substitute from your type mineral lists.

- Eat the right foods 80-90% of the time and the *Food Guide* will work for you.

- You may have allergies to wheat, corn, other grains, sugar, alcohol, and milk (examine your body reactions to these foods for fatigue, sinusitis, joint pain, skin rash, and gastro-intestinal reactions). Note that the *atrophic* type *requires* dairy foods for health and healing.

- Living out of a health food store is unnecessary (although such foods are healthier for you). If you want dietary perfection in your healing efforts, eat organic foods (from a health food store).

In addition to your body type needs other holistic healing matters also need your attention. I suggest that you refer to my web site and earlier books for that information: *DrStenbeck.net*

———

Nitorpheric Food Guide

[Superimpose the nutritional information from your Type Chapter into this Food Guide.]

Breakfast

FRUIT *salad, fresh (with citrus fruit) and* <u>*protein:*</u> *yogurt, kefir, milk, cheeses, or raw seeds or nuts* — *3+ times/week; or*

CEREALS *(whole grain), fruit, seeds, and nuts as desired* — *2+ times/week; or*

EGGS *(1-2) with lettuce, tomato, veges, non-wheat toast* — *0-3 times/week; or*

OTHER *choices* — *0-1 times/week*

<u>*Daily Liquids*</u>

Coffee, teas — *0-1 cups*
Pure water, citrus, fruit, or vegetable juices, soups, other — *as desired*
Wheat is a common allergy: avoid white breads; eat sour dough, millet, or oat breads instead.
Note: For in-between snacks, have fruit or vegetables, with seeds or nuts.

Food Guide
<u>Lunch</u>

SALADS, mixed green, with <u>protein</u> (cheese, soy, seeds, egg, etc.) Dressing: virgin olive oil and vinegar, low-fat dressings — 3-5 times weekly; and/or

VEGETABLES with salad (and a <u>protein</u>: yogurt, cottage cheese...) — 1-3 times/week; or

FRUIT salad (like breakfast)
*   — 1-2 times/week; or*

SANDWICH, whole grains, cheese and /or other non-flesh <u>protein</u>; small salad
*   — 0-2 times/week; or*

OTHER choices
*   — 0-1 times/week*

* Other oils less ideal; soybean oil is a common allergen; minimize commercial dressings.

Food Guide
Dinner

VEGETARIAN meals: include legumes, tofu, cheese, cottage cheese, seeds, nuts, egg, etc. (and/or salad) — *2+ times/week; or*

POULTRY/FISH (3-6 oz.), salad and/or vegetables — *0-2 times/week; or*

WHOLE GRAIN PASTA, cooked (barley, rice, millet, etc.), and salad/or vegetables — *0-2 times/week; or*

OTHER choices — *1-2 times weekly*

DESSERTS: Fruits, fresh or low-sugar desserts — as desired

Note: Be sure to include one or more selections from your type food lists in your daily food intake.

Note. Substitute flesh proteins with seeds, nuts, legumes, and other vegetables if *vegetarian.* You are vulnerable to being protein deficient so be careful to eat sufficient proteins and/or include a daily protein drink!

Food Guide Notes

Steamed Vegetables — Minerals are lost in the boiling of vegetables, so steaming or wok cooking is best.

Food Combinations — Eating proteins at the same meal with starches often results in indigestion, gas or constipation (as does eating fruit and starch together). For those of you with weak digestive systems, watch how this or other inharmonious combinations may be affecting you.

Periodic Detox Dieting — If you over-indulge in acid-ash foods, you need occasional elimination diets for tissue waste-acid removal, supervised by a nutritional doctor.

Minimize —
- Plums, cranberries, and their juices
- Commercial, sugared, and fatty salad dressings
- Red meats, processed meats, wines, alcohol, and milk
- Coffee, white sugar, fructose, and chemical sugar substitutes
- Exposure to drugs, environmental chemicals, pesticides
- Avoid eating allergic foods

Healthy Weight — You have a good ability to lose and control weight by following the Food Guide instructions. If you gain weight, the most common reason is liver or kidney irritation due to food allergies or negative emotions—the key is to eat non-allergic foods. The *atrophic and marasmic* types usually need to gain weight. (Obviously, if you have a medical condition that contradicts this advice, do not change your diet!)

———

In Conclusion

It is difficult to discern some *Thin* types from *Muscle* types (like the lean and strong *calciferic, nervimotive, and medeic* types). Study them well and you will see the differences.

———

Appendix

Brief Extracts from
<u>The 22 Unique Body Types</u>

A. Types / Minerals   56
B. Researchers   61
C. Genetics, Types, and Diet   63
D. Help identifying your body type,
   with Dr. Stenbeck   66
E. On-line Health Consultation   69
   with Dr. Stenbeck
F. Notes   70

Appendix A

Types
(Brief extract)

Type comes from 'typus' meaning an image or impression, the study of types being called typology.

▶ *Rocine: "A combination of mental and structural features is consistently found in people of the same type."*

Rocine wrote that all types are69

a mixture of positive and negative qualities. He based his work on the biochemical individuality of our *mineral* absorption and utilization. Of course, all minerals are absorbed, but he postulated that different types of people *selectively* absorb certain minerals, to a greater or lesser extent, requiring specific mineral foods for their enhanced health and healing. This is the basis of his types.

▶ *The type information cannot predict what or who you will become, or how successful or not, but your type is capable of bringing a creative excellence to whatever you do in life. If your type has negative qualities that you disagree with, remember that they are only tendencies and may or may not manifest in you.*

This book enlarges on Rocine's premise (early 1900's), integrated with the later research of Herbert Sheldon, M.D., Ph.D., at Harvard University (1930's), along with my fifty years of observations and experience with this subject.

Comparing your shared physical (and sometimes psychological) descriptions with the Celebrity Lists further assists the identification of your type. It is not that you will look exactly like, or be a twin to, any particular celebrity. Look closely at a celebrity's features: face, profile, height, weight, head, etc. If you know something about their talents, beliefs, success and failure spheres, health and weight challenges, attitudes and behaviors, etc., then you get clues as to what your type may be.

Understanding Types and Sub-Types

Each of us has a clearly discernible dominant type. Visualize the celebrity examples from movies, politics, sports, the arts and public life, and try to identify with their physical features. Look for similar features, remembering that you will not recognize all attributes in yourself. You are not looking for your twin!

The sub-type issue is the main reason people of the same major type can look so different. Remember that a type description does not characterize you exactly, but depicts your individual variant of a type.

▶ *The type questionnaire pinpoints the major features of that type: if the celebrity examples are unhelpful, you may be an unusual variant (in which case ignore the celebrity issue and give yourself 7 points on Question 1).*

―――――

Minerals

Minerals are essential life nutrients that accelerate enzyme and chemical reactions and provide a basis for your body typing. Although found in all tissues, different minerals tend to be concentrated in certain organs, their presence or absence contributing to the healing of such tissues; e.g., zinc accelerates prostate healing; calcium and manganese promote bone, joint and connective tissue healing.

Specific foods nurture each type, some people needing meats for their health others needing a vegetarian diet. A high potassium diet nurtures one person, while another needs high sulfur, calcium, zinc, or another mineral.

Mineral Digestion and Absorption

Compared to vitamins, minerals are *difficult* to digest, absorb, and utilize. In people with strong digestive systems, this aspect may not be important. The following factors should be in place for optimal mineral metabolism:

1. Stomach Hydrochloric Acid Production
2. Parathyroid Hormone Balance
3. Organ Toxic Metal and Chemical Removal
   [See details in The 22 Unique Body Types.]

_____

Total Body Healing

Note that from a holistic healing perspective, in addition to minerals and type information, the following healing factors are necessary:

Nutrient Balance
Mental Balance
Emotional Balance
Spiritual Balance
Detoxifying Integrity

The above factors are all important to your total healing especially if you are interested in self-healing (see my earlier books).

———

Appendix B

Researchers
(Brief extract)

The predominant workers in this area of human individuality from around 1880's to the 1960's are Herbert Sheldon, M.D., Ph.D., Roger Williams, Ph.D., and Victor Rocine, D.Sc.

Much information on Sheldon's research exists on-line and in medical psychology libraries; for interested readers there are other lines of research published in the last century. This present book is primarily about Rocine's body types.

Herbert Sheldon M.D., Ph.D.

In contrast to Rocine, Sheldon at Harvard University in the 1930's was trained in the scientific method and did painstaking research and publishing on human individuality. In comparing his findings with Rocine's work, a direct putative correlation is visible.

Roger J. Williams, Ph.D.

Another significant researcher in human individuality is the renowned scientist and biochemist, Roger J. Williams. He demonstrated that different people have varying levels of nutrients, enzymes, and other metabolic chemicals in their bloodstreams.

▶ *Williams's research firmly expands on the premise of individual nutritional needs in human beings. If interested in his research, I highly recommend his book <u>Biochemial Individuality</u>.*

Victor Rocine, D.Sc.

Note that when a negative feature is indicated, say neurotic tendencies, all members of the type are <u>not</u> that way; it is a type tendency reported by Rocine.

Rocine studied type-related diseases finding links between mineral and dietary factors with individual types and their diseases. In each body type, one or more dominant minerals are preferentially absorbed and utilized over other minerals.

He recognized discrete body types from their physical appearance finding genetically based mineral dominance to be the determining feature. He also correlated their physical features with psychological characteristics.

———

Appendix C

Genetics, Types, and Diet
(Brief extract)

This section deals with how nervous system genetics helps determine your eating choices for health: you are either born to be a predominant meat eater, a partial or complete vegetarian, or something between the two. The genetic factor determining this dietary aspect is the *sympathetic and parasympathetic* components of your central nervous system. This represents a basic factor in eating for health.

This chapter helps you understand your dietary inheritance, although instinctively, you may already have arrived there!

- If born *sympathetic* dominant you are *genetically acid*, desiring a predominantly *vegetarian* diet for your health (about 70% fruit, salad, vegetables to 30% proteins and carbohydrates).

- If born *parasympathetic* dominant you are *genetically alkaline*, desiring a predominantly *carnivorous* diet for your health (about 70% proteins, carbohydrates to 30% fruits, salads, vegetables). Few of you ever choose to become vegetarian because of the difficulty in satisfying your protein needs without meats.

- If born ***intermediate*** dominant you may eat food groups with little concern for the acid/alkaline factor. However, after age 40, you need a semi-vegetarian diet for healthy eating.

———

Chart of Relative Nervous System Dominance

In the following Chart, if you relate to many of the symptoms on one side you probably have that nervous system dominance; relating to both sides indicates *Intermediate* dominance.

If Vegetarian (Over-acid)
Eat 70% fruits, salads, vegetables
And 30% proteins, carbohydrates

If Carnivore (Over-alkaline)
Eat 70% proteins, carbohydrates
And 30% fruits, salads, vegetables

If Intermediate
Eat 50:50 of acid and alkaline-ash foods

Make an *approximate* estimate of your daily acid and alkaline food intake (such ratios varying from type to type).

———

Symptoms of Relative Genetic Dominance

Vegetarians (Over-acid)	Carnivores (Over-alkaline)
Sympathetic Dominance	Parasympathetic Dominance
little or no flesh desire	desire flesh
easily constipated	rarely constipated
slow digestion	fast digestion
easily dehydrated	not dehydrated
strong thirst	low thirst
pale face	flushed face
high pulse after food	slow pulse after food
easy gag reflex	slow gag reflex
cool dry skin	moist warm skin
nervous stomach	calm stomach
little eyelid blinking	much blinking
nervous tendency	mostly calm
slower healing	faster healing
low oxygen-uptake	good oxygen-uptake
easily breathless	seldom breathless
insomnia common	sleep easier
few muscle cramps	some night cramps
calcium deposits rare	get calcium deposits

Appendix D

Help Identifying your Body Type with Dr. Stenbeck

If you desire help in identifying your body type, follow these instructions, and answer the questionnaire. For further information and fees, send me an email from page one of the website:

DrStenbeck.net

First name: _____

Country of birth: _____

Upload photos and send to the above website:

- Head and shoulders: front and side views

- Full body: front and side views

- Also 1-2 teenage views

- If possible, casual photos of mother, father, siblings

MY TYPE CLASS MAY BE: _____

   (Thin, Muscle, or Fat)

AGE   -   _____

HEIGHT -   _____ feet/inches

MY WEIGHT -   _____ pounds

- Heaviest at age: _____

- Lightest as adult: _____

- Estimate age 15: _____

VISION - Excellent Average   Poor:

HAIR - Natural color: _____

- Thin/thick? _____

- balding? _____

SKIN - Quality: _____

- History of acne, boils, other:

_____

_____

TEETH - Strong Weak Dentures

- Cavity history: Many Moderate Few

MUSCLES - Strong Average Weak

Sports played _____

JOINTS - Strong Average Weak

HEALTH - Childhood diseases?

_____

_____

- Adult diseases?

_____

AVERAGE DIET

- Beef _____ (times/week)

- Poultry _____ (times/week)

- Fish _____ (times/week)

- Eggs _____ (times/week)

- Water _____ (glasses/day):

- Vegetarian? Vegan? _____

- Other? _____

- Did your childhood diet differ? _____

The above will help me know who you are! I will send yo a follow-up questionnaire for further help in identifying your body type.

Appendix E

On-line Health Consultation with Dr. Stenbeck

For further information, or to comment on this book, or to receive a response on any health issue from a holistic viewpoint, send an email inquiry from page one of my website:

DrStenbeck.net

Following that, I will suggest further healing needs, which we may pursue with an on-line consult.

———

Appendix F

Notes

See my book *The 22 Unique Body Types,* available at the usual online source, for further information and details on all of the 22 Types. The Appendix in that book also has more information about:

- *Mineral Functions and Food Sources*

- *Further Reading*

———